Understanding Cancer of the Breast

3 Bath Place, Rivington Street, London, EC2A 3JR

BACUP was founded by Dr Vicky Clement-Jones, following her own experiences with ovarian cancer, and offers information, advice and emotional support to cancer patients and their families.

We produce publications on the main types of cancer, treatments, and ways of living with cancer. We also produce a newspaper, *BACUP News*, three times a year.

Our success depends on feedback from users of our services. We thank everyone, particularly patients and their families, whose advice has made this booklet possible.

Administration 071 696 9003   Charity Registration No. 290526
Cancer Information Service 071 613 2121
Freeline (outside London) 0800 181199
Counselling Service 071 696 9000 (London based)

Medical consultant: Maurice Slevin, MD, FRCP

Editor: Annie Jackson

Cover design by: Malcom Harvey Young

Illustrations by: Andrew Macdonald and Alexa Rutherford

BACUP thanks Patsy Ryan RGN for her work on revising and updating the test of this booklet.

First published 1986
3rd revised edition published 1991, reprinted 1993
©BACUP 1986, 1987, 1991

Typeset and printed in Great Britain by Lithoflow Ltd., London

ISBN 1-870403-43-6

Contents

Introduction

This information booklet has been written to help you understand more about breast cancer. We hope it answers some of the questions you may have about its diagnosis and treatment.

We can't advise you about the best treatment for yourself because this information can only come from your own doctor who is familiar with your full medical history.

At the end of the booklet you will see a list of other BACUP publications, some useful addresses and recommended books. If, after reading this booklet you think it has helped you, do pass it on to any of your family and friends who might find it interesting. They too may want to be informed so that they can help you cope with any problems you may have.

What is cancer?

The organs and tissues of the body are made up of tiny building blocks called cells. Cancer is a disease of these cells. Although cells in different parts of the body may look and work differently, most repair and reproduce themselves in the same way. Normally, this division of cells takes place in an orderly and controlled manner, but if, for some reason, this process gets out of control, the cells will continue to divide, developing into a lump which is called a tumour. Tumours can either be benign or malignant.

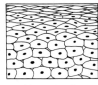
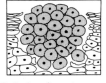

Normal cells   Cells forming a tumour

In a benign tumour the cells do not spread to other parts of the body and so are not cancerous. If they continue to grow at the original site, they may cause a problem by pressing on the surrounding organs or tissues.

A malignant tumour consists of cancer cells which have the ability to spread beyond the original site, and if left untreated may invade and destroy surrounding tissues. Sometimes cells break away from the original (primary) cancer and spread to other organs in the body via the bloodstream or lymphatic system. When these cells reach a new site they may go on dividing and form a new tumour, often referred to as a 'secondary' or a 'metastasis'. (If you have been told you have secondary breast cancer, BACUP has a booklet called *Understanding Secondary Breast Cancer* which we can send you.)

Doctors can tell whether a tumour is benign or malignant by examining a small sample of cells under a microscope.

It is important to realise that cancer is not a single disease with a single cause and a single type of treatment. There are more than 200 different kinds of cancer, each with its own name and treatment.

The breasts

The breasts are made up of fat, connective tissue and gland tissue which is divided into lobes. A network of ducts spreads from the lobes towards the nipple. When a woman is pregnant, the breasts produce milk to feed the baby.

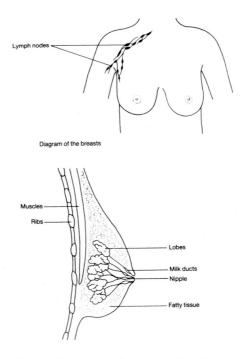

Diagram of the breasts

The breasts are seldom the same size as each other, and may feel different at different times of the menstrual cycle, sometimes becoming lumpy just before a period.

Under the skin, a 'tail' of breast tissue extends into the armpit (axilla). The armpits also house a collection of lymph glands which make up part of the lymphatic system. This is a network of lymph glands connected throughout the body by minute vessels called lymph vessels. A yellow fluid (lymph), containing cells called lymphocytes which are designed to fight disease, flows through the lymphatic system.

Breast tumours (lumps)

Nine out of ten breast lumps are benign and are not cancers. Most benign breast lumps are cysts. These are sacs of fluid which build up in the breast tissue. Another common benign breast lump is a fibroadenoma - a collection of fibrous glandular tissue. Benign breast lumps are easily treated if they are causing discomfort.

Men can develop breast cancer but it is one hundred times less common than in women.

If you do notice a lump in your breast, don't delay visiting your doctor. Anything unusual should always be examined, because even though most breast lumps are benign, they still need to be checked to rule out the possibility of cancer. Also, if it is cancer, the earlier the treatment, the better the chance of cure.

What causes breast cancer?

The causes of breast cancer are not yet completely understood but certain women do seem to be at a slightly higher risk of developing the disease. Women with a family history of breast cancer, particularly in their mother or sister, women who either have no children or had them late in life and women whose periods started when they were very young or whose menopause occurred late, all seem to run a slightly greater risk. There is some evidence to suggest that women who eat a diet high in animal fat may have a very slightly increased chance of developing breast cancer.

Some studies have shown that women who took the earlier types of the contraceptive pill (which contained more oestrogen than current pills) may have a slightly greater chance of developing breast cancer than women who have never taken the pill.

There is no evidence that damage to a breast (such as a knock) causes cancer.

What are the symptoms of breast cancer?

In ninety per cent of women, breast cancer is first noticed as a lump in the breast. There are, however, other signs to be aware of:

Breast: Change of size or shape
              Dimpling or flaking of the skin
              Lump or thickening

Nipple: Discharge (very rare)
              Rash on nipple or surrounding area (also very rare)
              Becomes inverted (turned in)
              Lump or thickening

Arm: Swelling of upper arm
              Swelling in armpit

Pain in your breast is not usually a symptom of breast cancer. In fact, many healthy women find their breasts feel lumpy and tender before a period, and some types of benign breast lumps are painful.

Early detection (screening)

The earlier breast cancer is diagnosed and treated, the better are the long-term prospects for women with the disease.

Breast self-awareness

Mammography (see below) can detect changes in the breast tissue before they develop into a lump large enough to be easily felt with the fingers. Nevertheless more than 90% of breast tumours are first detected by women themselves.

It is therefore important that you should become familiar with how your breasts normally feel, at different times of the month, by looking at and feeling them regularly during everyday activities like showering, bathing and dressing. You will then quickly be aware if there are any changes in your breasts that are not normal to you.

If you are concerned about anything unusual in your breasts — for example, in the size or outline shape of the breast, any puckering, dimpling or flaking of the skin, a lump or thickening in the breast, discharge from the nipple, or unusual pain or discomfort — you should make an appointment to discuss this with your doctor.

If you feel uncomfortable and anxious about feeling your breasts, you may find it helpful to discuss your worries with your doctor or nurse, or the staff at a well woman clinic. They will be able to reassure you about the changes you can normally expect to see in your breasts, and to advise you on the best way to become aware of how your breasts should look and feel.

BACUP has a leaflet on breast self-awareness which we would be happy to send you.

Mammography

Mammograms (breast X-rays) can often detect cancer before it can be felt, and for women over the age of 50, this is the best method of detection. The NHS offers mammograms to all women between the ages of 50 and 64, every three years, as part of a national breast-screening programme.

Some women have been concerned about having this type of regular screening, as each mammogram directly exposes the breasts to a small dose of X-rays. However, the tiny risk of these X-rays actually causing any harm is far outweighed by the benefits of detecting early breast cancer.

A screening programme for women younger than 50 is as yet of unproven value. Women who are not in the national screening age group and who have a family history of breast cancer can discuss with their doctor whether they should have regular screening. If you are too young for mammograms, ultrasound (see page 10) can be used instead if necessary.

You should remember that mammograms are not 100% foolproof. If, despite having a mammogram which showed no cancer, you find a lump in your breast, you should have it seen by a doctor immediately.

How does the doctor make the diagnosis?

You will probably begin by seeing your family doctor (General Practitioner) who will examine you and arrange any tests and X-rays you may need. Your GP may need to refer you to hospital for specialist advice or treatment.

At the hospital the doctor will take your medical history before doing a physical examination. Your doctor will examine your breasts and feel for any enlarged lymph nodes under your arms and at the base of your neck. A chest X-ray and blood test may also be taken to check your general health.

The following tests are all used to diagnose cancer of the breast and your doctor may arrange for you to have one or more of them at the hospital.

Mammography

This is an X-ray technique for examining the breasts. It is especially useful for detecting early changes in the breast when it may be difficult to feel a lump. Some women find mammography uncomfortable because pressure is put on the breasts, but this only lasts a few minutes.

Ultrasound

This test is painless and takes just a few minutes.

This test uses sound waves to build up a picture of the inside of the body. It is usually used for women under 35 whose breasts are too dense to give a clear picture with mammography. It is also used to see if a lump is solid or contains fluid (a cyst).

A special gel is spread onto the breasts and a small device, like a microphone, which emits sound waves, is passed over the area. The echoes are converted into a picture using a computer.

Needle aspiration

This is a quick simple procedure which is done in the outpatient clinic. Using a fine needle and syringe, the doctor takes a sample of cells from the breast lump and sends it to the laboratory to see if it contains any malignant cells.

Needle biopsy

This test uses a slightly larger needle than the one used for aspiration. It is done under a local anaesthetic which numbs the area and allows the doctor to take a biopsy which is a small piece of tissue from the lump. The sample is examined in the laboratory to check for signs of cancer.

Excision biopsy

In this biopsy the whole lump is removed under a general anaesthetic and sent to a laboratory for examination. This may mean an overnight stay in hospital but can be done as a day stay in some hospitals.

Further tests

If the tests show that you have breast cancer your doctor may want to do some further tests to see if there has been any spread of the disease. These help the doctor to decide on the best type of treatment for you. The tests may include any of the following.

Liver ultrasound scan

Ultrasound (see opposite) can be used to measure the size and position of any tumour. It is a painless test and only takes a few minutes. It will probably be done in the hospital scanning department.

You will be asked to lie on a couch. A gel will be spread on your abdomen and a small device like a microphone will be passed over the area. The echoes are converted into a picture using a computer.

Bone scan

For this test, a mildly radioactive substance is injected into a vein, usually in the arm. Abnormal bone takes up more radioactivity than normal bone. This radioactivity is picked up by the scanner.

This test does not make you radioactive and it is completely safe for you to be with children and other people afterwards.

Before you leave the hospital you will usually be given a follow-up appointment for about one to two weeks. This allows time for the laboratory results to come through. Obviously this waiting period will be an anxious time for you and it may help to talk about your worries with a partner, close friend or relative.

The stages of breast cancer

As well as detecting breast cancer, or confirming the doctor's initial diagnosis, the tests also show whether the cancer has spread. Breast cancer is divided into stages and these help doctors decide on the most appropriate treatment for the disease.

Stage one: The tumour measures under two centimetres, the lymph nodes in the armpit are not affected and the cancer has not spread elsewhere in the body.

Stage two: The tumour measures between two and five centimetres, or the lymph nodes are affected, or both, but the cancer has not spread further.

Stage three: The tumour is larger than five centimetres in size, lymph nodes are usually affected, but there has been no further spread.

Stage four: The tumour is of any size, lymph nodes are usually affected and the cancer has spread to other parts of the body. This is secondary breast cancer.

This booklet deals with the treatment of all stages of breast cancer, but BACUP has a separate booklet on secondary breast cancer which we can send you.

What types of treatment are used?

Surgery, radiotherapy, hormone therapy and chemotherapy may be used alone, or in combination, to treat breast cancer. Your doctor will plan your treatment by taking into consideration a number of factors, including your age, general health, the type and size of the tumour, what it looks like under the microscope and whether it has spread beyond the breast.

You may find that other women at the hospital are having different treatment from yourself. This will often be because their illness takes a different form, therefore they have different needs. It may also be because doctors take different views about treatment. If you have any questions about your own treatment don't be afraid to ask your doctor or hospital nurse. It often helps to make a list of the questions for your doctor and to take a close relative or friend with you to remind you of questions at the time, or the answers afterwards.

Some women find it reassuring to have another medical opinion to help them decide about their treatment. Most doctors will be pleased to refer you to another specialist for a second opinion if you feel this will be helpful.

Surgery

Your doctor will discuss with you the most appropriate type of surgery, depending on the size and any spread of the cancer. Before any operation make sure that you have discussed it fully with your doctor. It may help to make a list of any questions you have before your visit. Remember, no operation or procedure will be done without your consent.

If a diagnosis of breast cancer has already been made, either by needle aspiration or biopsy, the surgeon can discuss your operation with you in advance.

Sometimes a definite diagnosis can't be made before the operation and the surgeon will need to remove the lump so it can be examined under a microscope.

The lump is removed and examined later. If it is necessary, a further operation can be arranged for a few days afterwards. This allows you more time to prepare yourself.

In the past, the usual way of doing this operation involved removing the lump to be examined under a microscope while the patient was still under anaesthetic. To do this, the lump was frozen and this was, therefore, called a frozen section. If the lump was malignant and a further operation was necessary, the surgeon did it straight away. Nowadays, this is a rare procedure. Most surgeons agree a frozen section is of no more benefit than waiting a few days for the result, giving the woman more time to prepare herself if a mastectomy is necessary.

For many women it is now possible to have smaller operations rather than a mastectomy. All breast surgery, however, will leave some type of scar, and the cosmetic effect depends on the technique used. It is usually possible to discuss with the doctor or nurse beforehand what your breast will look like after surgery.

Lumpectomy

This is the removal of the breast lump together with some surrounding tissue. A lumpectomy is now possible for many women. It removes the least amount of breast tissue, but leaves a small scar and sometimes a small dent in the breast. For most women, the appearance of the breast after lumpectomy is good.

Segmentectomy

This is similar to a lumpectomy but as it involves removing more breast tissue it may be more noticeable, particularly in women who have small breasts. In women with large breasts it is usually less noticeable.

Mastectomy

For some women the most appropriate treatment is still a mastectomy (removal of the breast). A simple mastectomy removes only the breast tissue. A radical mastectomy also removes the muscles on the chest wall (this operation is now rare). A modified radical mastectomy removes the breast and lymph nodes often together with a small muscle from the chest wall.

Lymph gland removal

With any of these operations, the surgeon will usually remove lymph glands from under your arm. This is done to check whether any cancer cells have spread from the breast. Some doctors believe in removing all the armpit lymph glands, while others remove just a few lymph glands as a representative sample.

Breast reconstruction

It is often possible for women who have had a mastectomy to have their breast reconstructed. Sometimes this can be done at the same time as the mastectomy, but usually it is done some months, or even years after the original operation.

If you would like to consider breast reconstruction, discuss it with your doctor at the beginning of your treatment so that he or she can tell you about the different methods available.

BACUP has a booklet on breast reconstruction which we can send you.

After your operation

Your stay in hospital will depend on the extent of surgery you have had. You will be encouraged to get out of bed and start moving about as soon as possible after your operation. You may have a drainage tube in place from the wound. This will usually be removed a few days after the operation by the nurses on the ward.

After your operation you may have some pain or discomfort for a few days. There are several different types of painkilling drugs available which are very effective. If you do still have pain it is important to let the nurse looking after you know as soon as possible so that more effective painkillers can be prescribed.

After a lumpectomy or segmentectomy your stay in hospital will probably only be a few days. Women who have had a mastectomy usually stay in hospital for eight to ten days after their operation. After a mastectomy the arm on the affected side may feel stiff. You will probably be recommended to do simple arm exercises.

After a mastectomy you will be given a lightweight foam prosthesis (artificial breast) which you can put inside your bra. This is specially designed to be worn immediately after the operation when the area will be feeling tender. There are several types of prosthesis available on the NHS and the Breast Care and Mastectomy Association (BCMA) can supply you with a list of stockists throughout the country (see address on page 41).

Before you leave hospital you will be given an appointment to attend an outpatient clinic for your post-operative check up. This is a good time to discuss any problems you may have after your operation.

When you get home, do take things gently for a while. You may feel physically and emotionally exhausted so try to have plenty of rest and eat a well-balanced diet.

If the surgeon has removed lymph nodes from under your arm, or you have had radiotherapy (see page 20) to the armpit, your hand and arm are more vulnerable to infection. Even a small cut or a burn or graze can cause a flow of lymphatic fluid from other parts of the body, which will make the affected area swell and feel very sore. This is called lymphoedema. You should take great care of your hands, particularly for example when gardening, pruning roses, or playing with cats, and always wear rubber gloves when washing up, to reduce your risk of lymphoedema. If you do get any sign of swelling, pain or tenderness in your arm or hand, you should report it to your doctor straightaway. BACUP has a leaflet on lymphoedema which we can send you.

Living with breast surgery

Breast cancer surgery, whether it removes all your breast, or only a part of it, can be a deeply traumatic experience. You may feel that your breasts are very important to your idea of yourself as a woman and find that the alteration to your appearance severely affects your self-confidence. It is little wonder that the loss of a breast, or a part of a breast, has been compared to a bereavement, and women need time to come to terms with that loss.

All women find different ways of trying to come to terms with their altered bodies. Some prefer to see the results of the surgery for the first time alone. Others may want the support of a partner or close friend, or doctor or nurse, when they take their first look. Either way, the first months are likely to be very upsetting and many women are swamped with conflicting emotions. Grief, fear, shock, anger and resentment mixed, perhaps, with relief that the cancer has been found and treated – women have felt all or some of these to varying extents as they start to live with the effects of breast cancer surgery.

Help is available though. No woman has to deal with this experience alone, unless she prefers to do so. Many hospitals have specially trained breast nurse counsellors who are expert in supporting women at this time. Doctors, too, often have wide experience of helping women through this traumatic situation. The support of a caring partner or close friend can also be invaluable. The BCMA (see page 41) have an excellent nationwide volunteer support programme and can put you in touch with women in your area who have been through the same experience and who can offer comfort and practical advice.

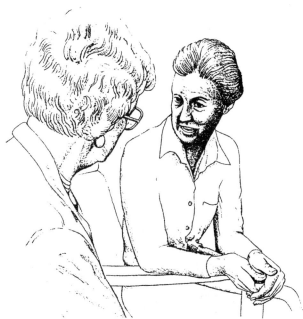

Although breast surgery will not affect your physical ability to have sex, it is obvious that the accompanying strong emotions may in some way alter your sexual feelings for a while. At any age, women need to feel relatively happy with their bodies to have a fulfilling sex life. Fear that a partner – even a long-standing one – may be put off by the result of the surgery can make women fearful of the moment they allow someone to see or touch their body.

There is no right or wrong time to take this step. When you do it, and the way you do it, depend entirely upon your own feelings and your relationships.

Some women feel so vulnerable, they need time simply to be alone to try to comfort themselves and build up the courage to face someone else – even a deeply loved partner. Others need almost immediate physical comfort and find loving touch a powerful relief to the fear of rejection. Letting someone else see their changed appearance is, for many women, the first step in coming to terms with their situation.

Again, you don't have to do this alone unless you prefer to do so. If undressing for bed with your partner on the first night home from hospital fills you with dread, you can try to lessen the impact. While you are still in hospital, the nurses can prepare your partner for how the operation site may look. A nurse, or your doctor, can even be with you both when you let your partner see the operation site. Alternatively, you may prefer a close relative or friend to be there and talk it over with you both afterwards.

Comforting words which may seem trite at first – such as, it will get better with time – are actually true. Although, if you have had a mastectomy, only a reconstruction operation will restore a breast, swelling will go down, bruising soon fades and scars will gradually become less obvious. As you become more used to the soft breast prosthesis, this will also help to restore your confidence.

This section has dealt mainly, and briefly, with the immediate emotional impact of breast cancer surgery. This is not meant to imply that in a few months you should feel fine and have fully accepted the changes to your body. The emotional rollercoaster often lasts longer: you may find all your anxieties returning each time you have to go for a follow-up appointment. New situations may bring fears, anger and insecurities flooding back; women without a partner, for example, may be particularly anxious if and when the time comes to get sexually involved with someone.

Help is not only available immediately after the operation. BACUP's face-to-face cancer counselling service is available in London to help anyone affected by cancer or we can put you in touch with trained counsellors in your area whom you can see at any time during or after your treatment. We also have up-to-date details of local support groups. Other national organisations which provide specific advice or support for women with breast cancer are listed on page 41, along with useful books.

The aftermath of breast cancer surgery can leave you emotionally and physically drained. Try to allow yourself to grieve for as long as you need and to enlist the caring support of others whenever and in whatever way is best for you.

Radiotherapy

Radiotherapy treats cancer by using high-energy rays to destroy the cancer cells, while doing as little harm as possible to normal cells. Two main types of radiotherapy are used to treat breast cancer; external radiotherapy and internal radiotherapy.

External radiotherapy

This is given as a course of treatment in the hospital radiotherapy department. Treatment is usually given from Monday to Friday with a rest at the weekend. The length of your treatment will depend on the type and size of the tumour and your doctor will discuss this with you. Whenever possible, treatment is given as an out-patient, but if you are already an in-patient you will be taken to the radiotherapy department each day from the ward.

For a few women, this type of radiotherapy is the only form of treatment needed to treat their breast cancer. More usually it is given as a back-up to surgery, after a lumpectomy, segmentectomy or mastectomy.

External radiotherapy does not make you radioactive and it is perfectly safe for you to be with other people, including children, after your treatment.

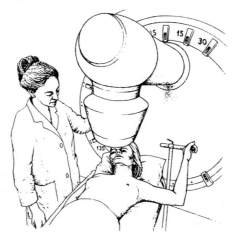

Planning your treatment

To ensure that you receive maximum benefit from your radiotherapy it has to be carefully planned. On your first visit to the radiotherapy department you may be asked to lie under a machine called a simulator which takes X-rays of the area to be treated. Treatment planning is a very important part of radiotherapy and it may take a few visits before the radiotherapist, the doctor who plans your treatment, is satisfied with the result.

Marks may be drawn on your skin to show the radiographer, who gives you the treatment, where the rays are to be directed. During the course of treatment this area should be kept as dry as possible to prevent the skin becoming sore and to keep the marks visible. Advice about skin care may vary from one hospital to another. Some departments will tell you not to wash the treatment area at all, for the time you are having treatment. Others will advise you to use only tepid water to wash the area, and then to dry it by patting gently with a soft towel. Do not rub the area, as this may make it sore. Perfumed soaps, talcs, deodorants, lotions and perfumes may also make your skin sore and should not be used.

Before radiotherapy is given the radiographer will position you carefully on the couch and make sure you are comfortable. During your treatment, which only takes a few minutes, you will be left alone in the room but you will be able to talk to the radiographer who will be watching you carefully from an adjoining room. Radiotherapy is not painful, but you do have to be still for several minutes while your treatment is being given.

Internal radiotherapy

This type of radiotherapy is sometimes given as a back-up after lumpectomy or segmentectomy. It is given by implanting wires containing a radioactive substance into the breast under a general anaesthetic. This gives an extra dose of radiation to the area surrounding the tumour. During this time you will need to stay in hospital and will be nursed in a separate room. The amount of time your visitors and the nursing staff can spend with you may be restricted to prevent them being unnecessarily exposed to radiation, and children and pregnant women will not be allowed to visit you at all. The radioactivity disappears once the wires are removed, and it is then perfectly safe for you to be with other people and children.

Side effects

Both external and internal radiotherapy to the breast sometimes cause side effects such as reddening and 'weepiness' of the skin, nausea and tiredness. These side effects gradually disappear once your course of treatment has finished though the tiredness may continue for some months. After a lumpectomy or segmentectomy, radiotherapy may make the breast feel firmer. It may also leave small red marks on the skin, which are due to tiny broken blood vessels. For many women, however, the cosmetic appearance of the breast is very good.

Can breast cancer be stopped from spreading?

The reasons why breast cancer may spread to other parts of the body are unknown as yet. The smaller the tumour, the less likely it is to spread. Sometimes, however, the cancer may already have released cells into the bloodstream or lymphatic system. If the lymph nodes in the armpit have been affected, there is a slightly increased risk that this will have happened.

Cancer cells carried in the bloodstream or lymphatic system can sometimes set up tiny cancers (metastases) elsewhere in the body. These may be so minute they can remain undetected for several years. The risk of this happening, however, can be reduced for some women if they are given additional treatment after the operation to remove the breast tumour. This extra treatment is called adjuvant therapy.

The most commonly used adjuvant therapy for women who have not yet had the menopause is chemotherapy (see page 24). However, recent studies have shown that stopping the ovaries from functioning (see below) may also be an effective treatment for premenopausal women, and some women would prefer this to adjuvant chemotherapy. For women who have had the menopause, most doctors recommend tamoxifen treatment (see below).

Unfortunately there is no absolute guarantee that these treatments will prevent cancer spreading, but adjuvant therapy does reduce the risk of any metastases developing.

Hormone therapy

Hormones are substances that occur naturally in the body and control the growth and activity of normal cells. The female hormones, oestrogen and progesterone, can also affect the growth of breast cancer cells. Hormone therapy for breast cancer consists, in effect, of anti-hormonal treatments to prevent female hormones working on breast cancer cells.

Hormone therapy is sometimes given to post-menopausal women immediately after surgery or radiotherapy as adjuvant therapy.

Tamoxifen is one of the most common hormone therapies. In simple terms, it works by preventing oestrogen from latching onto breast cancer cells and encouraging them to grow. Tamoxifen is taken as a daily tablet and causes few side effects. BACUP has leaflets on tamoxifen which we could send you.

Artificial forms of progesterone (the commonest ones are Provera and Megace) can be used if tamoxifen isn't working effectively.

For pre-menopausal women, removing the ovaries (which reduces the level of oestrogen in the body) can be an effective method of treatment. The ovaries are removed by a minor operation, or stopped from working by giving a low dose of radiotherapy to the area (see page 20). Unfortunately, removing the ovaries does bring on an early menopause which can be distressing, especially for a woman hoping to have more children. It also causes typical menopausal side effects like hot flushes, dry skin, anxiety and depression. The BACUP nurses can give practical advice on coping with these symptoms, as well as emotional support.

A new group of drugs (known as pituitary downregulators, or LHRH analogues) 'switch off' the ovaries, preventing them from producing oestrogen-stimulating hormone released by the brain. This has the same effect as removing the ovaries, or giving them radiotherapy, but is reversible. As a result, many doctors now recommend these drugs rather than operating, or radiotherapy.

Aminoglutethimide is a drug that prevents various tissues in the body producing a prehormone which develops into oestrogen. This is usually used for post menopausal women, as their ovaries have stopped producing oestrogen, but their adrenal glands still produce the prehormone. Aminoglutethimide may cause some side-effects, such as rash and drowsiness. This drug is more commonly used to treat secondary breast cancer and more details of this treatment are given in our booklet *Understanding Secondary Breast Cancer.*

Chemotherapy

Chemotherapy is the use of anti-cancer (cytotoxic) drugs to destroy cancer cells. They work by disrupting the growth and division of cancer cells. They can be used as adjuvant therapy after surgery or radiotherapy for women (especially pre-menopausal women) who may be at risk of developing a recurrence of the disease.

The drugs are sometimes given orally or, more usually, intravenously (by injection into a vein). Chemotherapy is given as a course of treatment usually lasting a few days. This is followed by a rest period of a few weeks which allows your body to recover from any side effects of the treatment. The number of courses you have will depend on the type of cancer you have and how well it is responding to the drugs.

Chemotherapy is sometimes given as an out-patient but at other times it may mean spending a few days in hospital.

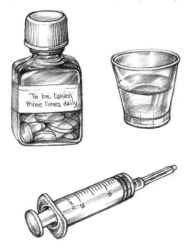

Side effects

While the drugs are acting on the cancer cells in your body they also reduce temporarily the number of normal cells in your blood. When these cells are reduced you are more likely to get an infection and you may tire easily. During chemotherapy your blood will be tested regularly and, if necessary, you will be given a blood transfusion or antibiotics.

Occasionally some patients may feel low spirited for a few days after their chemotherapy. Usually these feelings pass quite quickly, but if they persist, you should discuss this with your doctor.

Other side effects may include nausea, vomiting, diarrhoea and sometimes hair loss or thinning. Some drugs also make your mouth sore and cause small ulcers. Your doctor will prescribe regular mouthwashes and the nurse will show you how to do these properly. If you don't feel like eating meals you can supplement your diet with nutritious drinks. There is a wide range of these drinks available and you can buy them at most chemist shops. BACUP can send you a booklet called *Diet and the Cancer Patient* which gives helpful hints on overcoming eating problems. There is also now a new generation of drugs to stop you feeling sick (anti-emetics), which your doctor can prescribe for you, and which are very effective.

Although they may seem hard to bear at the time these side effects do disappear once your treatment is over. If you lose your hair it will grow back surprisingly quickly, and many people wear wigs, hats or scarves in the meantime. Most patients are entitled to a free wig from the National Health Service and your doctor or the nurses on the ward will be able to arrange this for you. BACUP has a free booklet called *Coping With Hair Loss* which we could send you.

Not all drugs cause the same side effects and some people have no side effects at all. Your doctor will tell you what problems, if any, to expect from your treatment.

It is important to remember that chemotherapy affects different people in different ways. Many people lead a normal life during their treatment while others find that they become very tired and have to take things more slowly.

BACUP also has a comprehensive booklet on chemotherapy which we could send you free of charge.

Can I still have children?

In the past doctors have been worried that if a woman who had had breast cancer became pregnant, the hormonal changes of pregnancy – particularly the increase in the hormone oestrogen – might make the cancer worse, or stimulate metastases. Recent research, however, seems to suggest that this is not the case, and that pregnancy does not make a recurrence of the disease more likely.

If you do want to have a child, you and your partner should discuss this with your doctor, who knows your full medical history, and talk over the risks and implications. It would be advisable to wait a while after your initial treatment has finished before trying to become pregnant. The longer you remain free of disease, the less likely it is that the cancer will recur; but you should probably consider carefully what might happen if, after having a baby, the cancer did come back, and whether you are both prepared to take the risk of that extra responsibility.

Unfortunately, women who have had radiotherapy to their ovaries, an operation to remove their ovaries or some types of chemotherapy will no longer be able to have children.

This added blow can be very hard for some women to live with – whether or not they already have children. Fertility is a very important part of many people's lives and not being able to have children can seem especially hard when you are already having to cope with cancer. Some people find it helpful to talk through their feelings about this distressing situation. BACUP can put you in touch with trained counsellors in your area, as can other organisations listed at the back of this booklet. We also have our own face-to-face counselling service based in London (the number is on page 40).

Loss of fertility is not usually something people can come to terms with in a short time. Allow yourself time to adjust to it and to express your sadness that a part of your life and a natural function of your body has been denied you. When you feel ready, talking with your partner, family or close friend may help you cope. Don't be afraid to ask your doctor for professional help. This is in no way a failure. People will understand that, whatever your circumstances, infertility is a situation with which most people cannot easily cope alone.

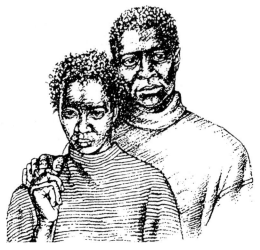

Contraception and hormone replacement therapy

As the cancer may be affected by hormones, women who have had breast cancer are usually advised not to take the contraceptive pill. The same advice is usually given about hormone replacement therapy. Recently there has been some evidence to suggest that giving the combined oestrogen and progesterone pill may be less likely to cause any problem than oestrogen alone. If you are having problems with menopausal symptoms, you may want to discuss this with your doctor.

Barrier methods of contraception such as condoms or the cap are suitable. KY jelly and baby oil (available without prescription from the chemist) are completely safe to use with barrier contraceptives if extra moisture is needed during sex.

Your hospital doctor can give you good contraceptive advice, as can your GP, who can also fit you for a cap if this is the contraceptive you choose. Coils (IUDs) are also effective – but not the ones that work by secreting progesterone, another female hormone. Again, your GP can fit you with a coil if you wish. Some women choose to be sterilised to prevent the risk of pregnancy.

The choice of an effective contraceptive is largely a personal one. Your likes and dislikes, and those of your partner if you have one, are obviously important. Some women also have religious and moral implications to consider. Unfortunately, the withdrawal and rhythm methods of contraception are not safe enough to be effective as protection against pregnancy in this case. Some women find that, if necessary, talking through their situation with their religious leader, or a trained counsellor, helps them find acceptable alternatives.

Follow up

After your treatment has been completed your doctor will want you to have regular check-ups and X-rays. These will often continue for several years. If you have any problems or notice any new symptoms in between these times, let your doctor know as soon as possible.

For more information about radiotherapy, chemotherapy, coping with hair loss, diet hints, tamoxifen, lymphoedema, breast reconstruction and secondary breast cancer, see our list of BACUP publications at the back of this booklet.

Research – clinical trials

Research into new ways of treating breast cancer is going on all the time. As no current cancer treatment results in the cure of all the patients treated, cancer doctors (oncologists) are continually looking for new ways to treat the disease and they do this by using clinical trials.

If early work suggests that a new treatment might be more effective than the standard treatment, cancer doctors will carry out trials to compare the new treatment with the current ones. Often several hospitals around the country take part in these trials.

The usual way cancer doctors carry out these trials is by comparing the new treatment with the best available standard treatment. This is called a controlled clinical trial and is the only way of scientifically testing a new treatment.

So that the treatments may be accurately compared, the type of treatment a patient receives is decided at random by a computer and not by the doctor treating the patient. This is because it has been shown that if a doctor chooses the treatment, or offers a choice to the patient, he or she may unintentionally bias the result of the trial.

In a randomised controlled clinical trial, half the patients will receive the best standard treatment and the other half will receive the new treatment, which may or may not prove to be better than the standard treatment. A treatment is deemed to be better either because it is more effective against the tumour or because it is equally effective and has the advantage of fewer unpleasant side effects.

The reason why your doctor would like you to take part in a trial (or study as they are sometimes called) is because until the new treatment has been tested scientifically in this way, it is impossible for doctors to know which is the best one to choose for their patients.

Your doctor must have your informed consent before entering you into any clinical trial. This means that you know what the trial is about, you understand why it is being conducted and why you have been invited to take part, and the treatment has been discussed with you.

Even after agreeing to take part in a trial, you can still withdraw at any stage if you change your mind. Your decision will in no way affect your doctor's attitude towards you. If you choose not to take part or you withdraw from a trial, you will then receive the best standard treatment rather than the new one with which it is being compared.

If you do choose to take part in these trials, it is important that whatever treatment you receive will have been carefully researched in preliminary studies, before it is fully tested in any randomised controlled clinical trial. By taking part in a trial you will be helping to advance medical science and thus improve prospects for patients in the future.

Your feelings

Most people feel overwhelmed when they are told they have cancer. Many different emotions arise which can cause confusion and frequent changes of mood. You might not experience all the feelings discussed below or experience them in the same order. This does not mean, however, that you are not coping with your illness. Reactions differ from one person to another – there is no right or wrong way to feel. These emotions are part of the process that many people go through in trying to come to terms with their illness. Partners, family members and friends often experience similar feelings and frequently need as much support and guidance in coping with their feelings as you do.

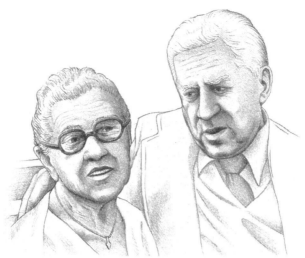

Shock and disbelief

'I can't believe it' 'It can't be true'

This is often the immediate, reaction when cancer is diagnosed. You may feel numb, unable to believe what is happening or to express any emotion. You may find that you can take in only a small amount of information and so you have to keep asking the same questions over and over again, or you need to be told the same bits of information repeatedly. This need for repetition is a common reaction to shock. Some people may find their feelings of disbelief make it difficult for them to talk about their illness with their family and friends, while others feel an overwhelming urge to discuss it with those around them; this may be a way of helping them to accept the news themselves.

Fear and uncertainty

'Am I going to die?' 'Will I be in pain?' 'Will the cancer come back?'

Cancer is a frightening word surrounded by fears and myths. One of the greatest fears expressed by almost all newly-diagnosed cancer patients is: 'Am I going to die?'

In fact, nowadays many cancers are curable if caught at an early enough stage. This is especially true of breast cancer.

Even if the cancer is not completely curable, modern treatments often mean that the disease can be controlled for years and many patients can live an almost normal life.

'Will I be in pain?' and 'will any pain be unbearable?' are other common fears. In fact, many cancer patients experience no pain at all. For those who do, there are many modern drugs which are very successful at relieving pain or keeping it under control.

Many people are anxious about their treatment; whether or not it will work and how to cope with possible side effects. It is best to discuss your individual treatment in detail with your doctor. Make a list of questions you may want to ask and don't be afraid to ask your doctor to repeat any answers or explanations you don't understand. You may like to take a close friend or relative to the appointment with you. If you are feeling upset they may be able to remember details of the consultation which you might have forgotten or you may want them to ask some of the questions you don't want to ask. Some people are afraid of the hospital itself. It can be a frightening place, especially if you have never been in one before, but talk about your fears to your doctor; he or she should be able to reassure you.

You may find the doctors can't answer your questions fully, or that their answers sound vague. It is often impossible to say for certain that they have got rid of the cancer completely. Doctors know from past experience approximately how many people will benefit from a certain treatment. It is impossible to predict the future for individual people. Many people find this uncertainty hard to live with; not knowing whether or not you are cured can be disturbing.

Uncertainty about the future can cause a lot of tension, but fears are often worse than the reality. Fear of the unknown can be terrifying so finding out about your illness can be reassuring. Discussing it with your family and friends can help to relieve tension caused by unnecessary worry.

Denial

'There's nothing really wrong with me' 'I haven't got cancer'

Many people cope with their cancer by not wanting to know anything about their cancer, or not wanting to talk about it. If that's the way you feel, then just say quite firmly to the people around you that you would prefer not to talk about your illness, at least for the time being.

Sometimes, however, it is the other way round. You may find that it is your family and friends who are denying your illness. They appear to ignore the fact that you have cancer, perhaps by playing down your anxieties and symptoms or deliberately changing the subject. If this upsets or hurts you because you want them to support you by sharing what you feel, try telling them how you feel. Start perhaps by reassuring them that you do know what is happening and that it will help you if you can talk to them about your illness.

Anger

'Why me of all people and why right now?'

Anger can hide other feelings such as fear or sadness. You may take your anger out on those who are closest to you and on the doctors and nurses who are caring for you. If you have a religious faith you may feel angry with your god.

It is understandable that you may be deeply upset by many aspects of your illness and you should not feel guilty about your angry thoughts or irritable moods. Relatives and friends though may not always realise that your anger is really directed at your illness and not against them. If you can, it may be helpful to tell them this at a time when you are not feeling quite so angry. If you find that difficult, perhaps you could show them this section of the booklet. If you are finding it difficult to talk to your family it may help to discuss the situation with a trained counsellor or psychologist. BACUP can give you details of how to get this sort of help in your area.

Blame and guilt

'If I hadn't .... this would never have happened'

Sometimes people blame themselves or other people for

their illness, trying to find reasons for why it should have happened to them. This may be because we often feel better if we know why something has happened. As doctors rarely know exactly what has caused your cancer though, there's no reason for you to blame yourself.

Resentment

'It's all right for you, you haven't got to put up with this'

Understandably, you may be feeling resentful and miserable because you have cancer while other people are well. Similar feelings of resentment may crop up from time to time during the course of your illness and treatment for a variety of reasons. Relatives too can sometimes resent the changes that the patient's illness makes to their lives.

It is usually helpful to bring these feelings out into the open so that they can be aired and discussed. Bottling up resentment can make everyone feel angry and guilty.

Withdrawal and isolation

'Please leave me alone'

There may be times during your illness when you want to be left alone to sort out your thoughts and emotions. This can be hard for your family and friends who want to share this difficult time with you. Reassure them that although you may not feel like discussing your illness at the moment, you will talk to them about it when you are ready.

Sometimes depression can stop you wanting to talk. It may be an idea to discuss this with your GP who can prescribe a course of antidepressant drugs or refer you to a doctor who specialises in the emotional problems of cancer patients. It is common for women with breast cancer to feel depressed, so there is no need to feel you are not coping if you ask for help.

Learning to cope

After any treatment for cancer it can take a long time to come to terms with your emotions. Not only do you have to cope with the knowledge that you have cancer but also the physical effects of the treatment.

The treatment for breast cancer can cause unpleasant side effects but some women do manage to lead an almost normal life during their treatment. Obviously you will need to take time off for your actual treatment and some time afterwards to recover. Just do as much as you feel like and try to get plenty of rest.

Don't see it as a sign of failure if you have not been able to cope on your own. Once other people understand how you are feeling they can be more supportive.

What to do if you are a friend or relative

Some families find it difficult to talk about cancer or share their feelings. It may seem best to pretend that everything is fine, and carry on as normal, perhaps because you don't want to worry the patient or feel you are letting her down if you admit to being afraid. Unfortunately, denying strong emotions like this can make it even harder to talk together, and lead to the patient feeling very isolated.

Partners, relatives and friends can help by listening carefully to what, and how much the woman wants to say. Don't rush into talking about the illness. Often it is enough just to listen and let her talk when she is ready.

Whether you are the woman with breast cancer or her partner, close relative or friend, look out for people with a positive attitude, as they are always more helpful than the pessimistic ones.

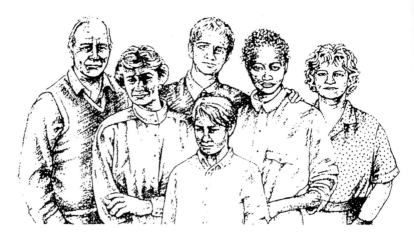

Talking to children

Deciding what to tell children about cancer is difficult. How much you tell them will depend upon their age and how grown up they are. Very young children are concerned with immediate events. They don't understand illness and need only simple explanations of why their relative or friend has had to go into hospital. Slightly older children may understand a story explanation in terms of good cells and bad cells but all children need to be repeatedly reassured that the illness is not their fault because, whether they show it or not, children often feel they may somehow be to blame and may feel guilty for a long time. Most children of about 10 years old and over can grasp fairly complicated explanations.

Adolescents may find it particularly difficult to cope with the situation because they feel they are being forced back into the family just as they were beginning to break free and gain their independence. Daughters in particular may worry that their mother's illness can be passed on to them.

An open, honest approach is usually the best way for all children. Listen to their fears and be aware of any changes in their behaviour. This may be their way of expressing their feelings. It may be better to start by giving only small amounts of information and gradually building up a picture of the illness. Even very young children can sense when something is wrong so don't keep them in the dark about what is going on. Their fears of what it might be are likely to be far worse than the reality.

What you can do

Many people feel helpless when they are first told they have cancer and think there is nothing they can do, other than hand themselves over to doctors and hospitals. This is not so. There are many things you, and your family, can do at this time.

Understanding your illness

If you and your family understand your illness and its treatment you will be better prepared to cope with the situation. In this way you at least have some idea of what you are facing.

For information to be of value though it must come from a reliable source to prevent it causing unnecessary fears. Personal medical information should come from your own doctor who is familiar with your medical background. As mentioned earlier it can be useful to make a list of questions before your visit or take a friend or relative with you to remind you of things you want to know but can forget so easily. Other sources of information are given at the end of this booklet.

Practical and positive tasks

At times you may not be able to do things you used to take for granted. But as you begin to feel better you can set yourself some simple goals and gradually build up your confidence. Take things slowly and one step at a time.

Many people talk about 'fighting their illness'. This is a healthy response and you can do it by becoming involved in your illness. One easy way of doing this is by planning a healthy, well-balanced diet. Another way is to learn relaxation techniques which you can practise at home with tapes. Contact BACUP for more information.

Many people find it helpful to take some regular exercise. The type of exercise you take, and how strenuous, depends on what you are used to and how well you feel. Set yourself realistic aims and build up slowly.

If the idea of changing your diet or taking exercise does not appeal to you, do not feel you have to do it; just do whatever suits you. Some people find pleasure in keeping to their normal routine as much as possible. Others prefer to take a holiday or spend more time on a hobby.

Who can help?

The most important thing to remember is that there are people available to help you and your family. Often it is easier to talk to someone who is not directly involved with your illness. You may find it helpful to talk to a breast care nurse specialist, who is specially trained to offer support and advice. The BACUP nurses are also happy to discuss any problems about your breast cancer, and let you know of sources of support in your area (see page 40); others take comfort in talking to a religious leader.

There are several other people who can offer support in the community. District nurses work closely with GPs and make regular visits to some patients and their families at home. In many areas of the country there are also Macmillan and Marie Curie nurses, who are specially trained to look after people with cancer in their own homes. Let your GP know if you are having any problems so that proper home care can be arranged.

Some hospitals have their own emotional support services with specially trained staff and many of the nurses on the ward have training in counselling as well as being able to give advice about practical problems. The hospital social worker is also often able to help in many ways including counselling and giving information about social services and other benefits you may be able to claim while your are ill. For example, you may be entitled to meals on wheels, a home help or hospital fares. The social worker may also be able to help arrange childcare during and after treatment and, if necessary, help with the cost of childminders.

But there are people who require more than advice and support. They may find that despite their best efforts, the impact of cancer leads to depression, feelings of helplessness and anxiety. Specialist help in coping with these emotions is available in some hospitals. Ask your hospital doctor or GP to refer you to an expert in the special emotional problems of cancer patients and their relatives.

Sick pay and benefits

If you are employed, and unable to work, your employer will pay your first twenty-eight weeks sick pay. If, after this period, you are still unable to work you can claim Invalidity Benefit from the DSS.

If you are unemployed and not fit to work you will need to switch from Unemployment Benefit to Sickness Benefit. To do this you should contact your local DSS office and arrange to send them regular sickness certificates from your doctor. If you are ill and not at work do remember to ask your family doctor for a medical certificate to cover the period of your illness. If you are in hospital ask the doctor or nurse for a certificate, which you will need to claim benefit.

If because of your illness, you are finding it difficult to manage on your income, you may be entitled to Income Support (previously called Supplementary Benefit) and in some circumstances, you may be able to claim additional benefits.

For full advice on all the benefits available to you, contact your local DSS, Citizens' Advice Bureau or Social Services office. Their addresses and telephone numbers are in the 'phone book. The DSS is listed under Health and Social Security and Social Services under individual boroughs.

BACUP's services

Cancer Information Service

This service is staffed by specially trained cancer nurses. If you ring or write to us, your phone call or letter will always be answered by a nurse who can give you information on all aspects of cancer and its treatment and who will offer practical and emotional support, whether you have cancer yourself, or are the friend or relative of someone with the illness. A computerised directory and a library of resources are used by the nurses to help provide information to anyone who enquires about treatment, research, support groups, therapists, counsellors, financial assistance, insurance, home nursing services and much more. The nurse can also send you any of our other booklets which might be helpful.

The Cancer Information Service is open to telephone enquiries from 10 am to 7 pm, Monday to Thursday, and until 5.30 pm on Friday. The number is 071 613 2121 if you are ringing from London. You can call the service free of charge from outside the 071 and 081 telephone districts on 0800 181199.

Cancer Counselling Service

Emotional difficulties linked to cancer are not always easy to talk about and are often hardest to share with those to whom you are closest. Trained counsellors use their skills to help people talk about their thoughts, feelings and ideas and perhaps untangle some of the difficulties and confusion that living with cancer brings.

BACUP runs a one-to-one counselling service based at its London offices which it is intended to develop nationwide. The Counselling Service can also give you information about counselling services in your area, and discuss with you whether counselling would be appropriate and helpful for you.

For more information about counselling, or to make an appointment with BACUP's Counselling Service, please ring 071 696 9000 between 10 am and 5 pm, Monday to Friday.

Other useful organisations

Breast Care and Mastectomy Association (BCMA)

15-19 Britten Street	65 Bath Street	511 Lanark Road
London	Glasgow	Edinburgh
SW3 3TZ	G2 2BX	EH14 5DQ
Tel: 071 867 1103	Tel: 041 353 1050	Tel: 039 458 5598

Gives emotional support and practical advice to women who have or fear they may have breast cancer. It has a national volunteer support service, a Helpline and a prosthesis fitting service with a selection of bras and swimwear in both the Edinburgh and London offices.

Women's Nationwide Cancer Control Campaign
Suna House
128/130 Curtain Road
London
EC2A 3AR
Tel: 071 729 2229

Offers information and advice on the screening and early detection of breast cancer.

CancerLink

17 Britannia Street	9 Castle Terrace
London	Edinburgh
WC1X 9JN	EH1 2DP
Tel: 071 833 2451	Tel: 031 228 5557

Resource centre for cancer self-help and support groups throughout Britain and a telephone information service on all aspects of cancer.

Cancer Aftercare and Rehabilitation Society (CARE)
21 Zetland Road
Redland
Bristol
BS6 7AH
Tel: 0272 427419

An organisation of cancer patients, relatives and friends who offer help and support. Branches throughout the country.

Cancer Relief Macmillan Fund
15-19 Britten Street
London
SW3 3TZ
Tel: 071 351 7811

Provides home care nurses through the Macmillan Service and financial grants for people with cancer and their families.

Marie Curie Cancer Care
28 Belgrave Square
London
SW1X 8QG
Tel: 071 235 3325

Runs centres throughout the UK and a community nursing service to give care to patients at home.

Tak Tent Cancer Support – Scotland
G Block
Western Infirmary
Glasgow
G11 6NT
Tel: 041 332 6699

Provides information, support and counselling for cancer patients, their relatives and professional staff involved in their care. Speakers are available for those interested in hearing about the work of Tak Tent.

Tenovus Cancer Information Centre
142 Whitchurch Road
Cardiff
CF4 3NA
Tel: 0222 691998

Provides a counselling and information service personally or over the 'phone.

The Ulster Cancer Foundation
40-42 Eglantine Avenue
Belfast
BT9 6DX
Tel: 0232 663439

Provides information on all aspects of cancer.

Details of family planning and well woman clinics are available at your doctor's surgery.

Recommended reading list

Faulder, Carolyn
The Women's Cancer Book
Virago, 1989 (ISBN 0860 68993 X)

Faulder, Carolyn
Always A Woman
Thorsons, 1992
(ISBN 0-7225-2643-1)

Clyne Rachel
Cancer: Your Life, Your Choice
Wellingborough, Thorsons Publishing Group, 1989
(ISBN 0-7225-21-030)

Kfir, Nira and Slevin, Maurice
Challenging Cancer: From Chaos to Control
Tavistock/Routledge 1991
(ISBN 0 415 06344 2)   *

* Williams, Chris and Sue
Cancer: A guide for patients and their families
Chichester, Wiley, 1986
(ISBN 0-471-91017-1)

Bryan, Jenny, Lyall, Joanna
Living with Cancer
Penguin 1987
(ISBN 0-14-009409-1)

Baum, M
Breast Cancer: The Facts
Oxford University Press, 1981
(ISBN 0 19261 7273)

* These books are now out of print but may be available from libraries.